THE 8 DAY GREEN SMOOTHIE CLEANSE

Lose up to 13 Pounds in 8 Days with 25 Delicious Recipes

by Francesca DiMarco

Copyright © 2015 by Bright Ideas Editoria Ltd.

First Printing: 2015
Bright Ideas Editorial
PO Box 4095
Crested Butte, CO 81224
https://www.facebook.com/brightideaseditoria

Disclaimer

Although the author and publisher have made every effort to ensure that the information in this book was correct at press time, the author and publisher do not assume and hereby disclaim any liability to any party for any loss, damage, or disruption caused by errors or omissions, whether such errors or omissions result from negligence, accident, or any other cause.

This book is not intended as a substitute for the medical advice of physicians. The reader should regularly consult a physician in matters relating to his/her health and particularly with respect to any symptoms that may require diagnosis or medical attention.

FREE DOWNLOAD

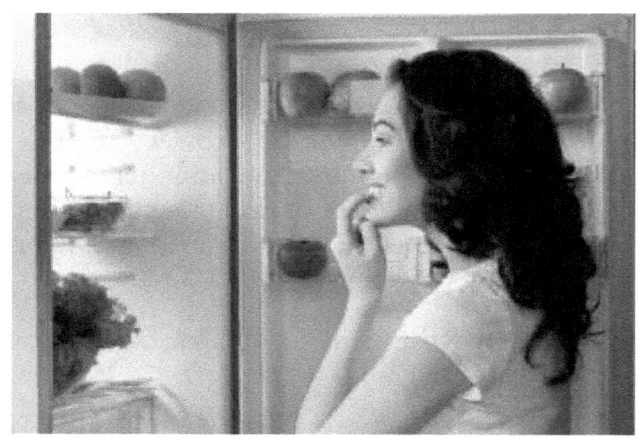

As a thank you for purchasing this book, I've created a free report full of healthy snack ideas, just for you!

FREE REPORT REVEALS 10 SCRUMPTIOUS SNACKS UNDER 200 CALORIES

"Smash the hangries with these skinny snacks (if your kids don't eat them first)"

You can download the free report at http://editoria.leadpages.net/snacks/

Table of Contents

Introduction: How I lost 13 Pounds in 8 Days

"I'm not losing weight. I'm getting rid of it. I have no intention of ever finding it again" Anonymous

When my oldest daughter turned a year old, my husband did an outrageous thing. He purchased a trip for two to Italy. I was completely freaked out. Not because I would be leaving my helpless toddler with my in-laws for ten days. They had raised four perfectly well-adjusted and happy adults and were my daughter's favorite people in the universe. These days I wouldn't dream of traveling without my kids. Now that they are old enough to appreciate new places and new experiences, I feel cheated when they aren't around. But when they were little, my motto was, "If they would have a better time with grandma, and I would have a better time if they were with grandma, they stay with grandma." So it wasn't the separation that freaked me out. It was the baby weight.

Italy is known for a lot of things: art, cars, wine, history, and lovers all come to mind. But the two things I was anticipating were clothes and food. There was no way I was going to a European fashion mecca and not shopping. I always buy my clothes on vacation. They are my souvenirs. Every time I put on something I bought on a trip, it brings back happy memories. And, as silly as this sounds when I say it out loud, I get a kick out of saying, "Oh, this? I got it in Rimini." I look for quality, things I can wear for years, and also value. There's not a label in my closet anyone would recognize. Well, except for Disney. But I knew I would want to shop, and I also knew I didn't want to shop for clothes that I could fit into at the time.

There are lots of diets that promise rapid weight loss. Atkins was the popular one at the time. But it didn't add up for me. The body needs the vitamins and minerals and fiber and energy that fruits and vegetables provide. I wasn't getting enough of them, and I knew it. Then my sister told me about a healthy shake she drank each morning, made from spinach, a banana, and some yogurt. I had my solution. The secret to rapid weight loss is in filling up the body with slow, healthy carbs, fats, fiber, and protein for long-lasting energy. My husband and I each replaced both breakfast and lunch with a fruit and vegetable smoothie with a little protein thrown in, and ate two small snacks and a dinner of lean proteins and more greens. We experimented with everything in our smoothies. Some of our recipes were delicious, and some, well, were not. But we drank them all, and it worked wonders. In the first eight days, I dropped 13 pounds, and I lost all 30 baby weight pounds before I boarded the plane. And I was *never hungry*. My husband lost several pant sizes but didn't weigh himself obsessively, so I can't put his progress into numbers.

It felt so good to feel sexy again. And it felt even better to shop. I bought cute skirts and strappy sandals, and sleek camisoles that showed off my tanned arms.

And I ate. Because I was in Italy. And then I drank a few more green smoothies when we got home. In fact, we both drink them regularly for a quick and healthy breakfast.

Chapter 1: Easy Does It

"You don't have to cook fancy or complicated masterpieces-just good food from fresh ingredients."
Julia Child

This book offers you the information you'll need to introduce green smoothies into your life. You will also learn the whys and the hows necessary to make the transition a smooth one. Be warned – green smoothies are totally addictive. Not only are they delicious, you will feel so energized and healthy after drinking them that you won't be able to image your life without them anymore. They are a fantastic way to lose weight quickly. Even after you have met your weight loss goals, green smoothies offer a fast and filling breakfast, and an excellent way to help meet your daily recommended quota of green vegetables.

If you are this far into this eBook, chances are you have a date circled in red on your calendar: the beginning of summer when the pools open; a tropical vacation; a wedding; a class reunion. There is a sense of urgency pumping through your body and your brain screaming, "Enough of this! I need to lose this weight now!" I applaud your initiative. This book will help you reach your goals. But I would like to caution you as well.

While it is entirely possible to lose 5, 10, or even 15 pounds in a week or two, most people who do so often gain back those same pounds within the next few months. This is because they use a weight loss system that is not sustainable. They sacrifice hard in the short term, and then when they reach their goal, they go right back to the behaviors that brought about the weight gain in the first place.

To avoid this very common pitfall, it is necessary to replace the old behaviors and habits with new ones that are just as satisfying as the old ones. Every single day cannot be a struggle. Every meal cannot be a sacrifice. If you feel overly restricted, at some point you will begin to rebel.

So don't overdo it. During the first week to 10 days, when smoothies are fresh and new, drink them as meal replacements for two of your three main meals, and include a couple of light, solid food snacks. Do not replace all three meals. For your third meal, include a portion of lean protein, and lots of whole healthy vegetables. Experiment with different preparations. Try roasting, grilling, and steaming your meals. Use lots of herbs for flavor. Eat big salads with fruits and colors. Make your third meal fun, something to look forward to. It doesn't need to be decadent to be delicious.

There are three important reasons for making sure that you eat at least one meal, if not two meals, a day. The first is that you will begin to miss the act of chewing and eating food very quickly. If food feels forbidden, you will fantasize about it, and then consume an extra-gargantuan double everything pizza and an entire cheesecake. It is human nature. The second reason is that, chances are, you are combining this weight loss plan with an increase of activity, and it is critical that you get the right amount of protein each day.

Protein can be exceptionally tricky. It is critical for building muscles when you exercise, for healthy hair and skin and nails, for strong bones, for producing the hormones and enzymes you use constantly. It also helps you to feel full longer. But many foods that contain protein can be high in saturated fat, so it is important to stick with lean proteins like fish, white meat, and legumes for weight loss and heart health. Also, extra protein doesn't get stored like fat does. If you consume more than you need, your body eliminates it. When the body breaks down protein to use it, uric acids forms in the blood. The kidneys are supposed to filter the uric acid out, but if there is more than the kidneys can handle, uric acid crystals build up on joints and form a type of arthritis called gout.

Gout flare-ups are exceptionally painful. The percentage of people with gout in both the US and the UK doubled from the 1960s to the 1990s, and it keeps rising every year. Researchers suspect it is due to the increase in high protein diets, and high protein drinks. Once a person contracts gout, there is no cure. All they can do is manage their diet and sometimes take medication to prevent flare-ups. My husband can tell you first-hand how difficult this can be. He developed gout in his early 30s after drinking too many high-protein workout recovery drinks. Every year he has at least one crippling gout episode. (Being a Jane Austen devotee, I made him go to Bath for the waters and so I could visit The Pump Room.)

How much protein, then, is the right amount? The Center for Disease Control in the US says that men should get 56 grams each day, and women should get 46 grams. To give you an idea of how much that is, a five-ounce portion of chicken breast, about half a breast, has roughly 30 grams. A three-ounce serving of beef has 21 grams. Eight ounces of yogurt has 11 grams. Eight ounces of milk has 8 grams. An ounce of nuts has about 9 grams. (If it bothers you that I am mixing ounces and grams, I sincerely apologize. It bugs me too, but that is how the nutritional content in the US is reported. Serving sizes are in ounces, and nutritional content is in grams. We still use calories, though, because we wouldn't want to get too metric-y). The CDC cautions that not more than one-third of your calories should come from protein. Be careful with adding protein powders to your smoothies. Read labels carefully and don't overdo it.

The last reason to make sure you eat at least one meal a day is that, though this may sound counter-intuitive, you need cooked vegetables too. Raw food aficionados will tell you that cooking destroys some of the vital nutrients found in your veggies. It does, to a certain extent. But it also *boosts* some of the benefits, especially many of the antioxidants. Just don't fry them.

Another note of caution: take care of your belly. Some people experience gastrointestinal issues when they go from a diet with very few vegetables to a diet rich in them. Blending the greens helps your body to process all of the insoluble fiber, but some people still have trouble. If you find yourself confined to the bathroom after your first green smoothie, you will need to work into it more gradually. You can also try reducing the green vegetable content of your smoothies and supplementing with more colorful veggies like carrots and beets. They tend to be higher in natural sugars, so careful with adding fruit as well, but they also tend to be higher in soluble fiber, and easier on the gut.

One last qualification: It is also important that you consult your physician before beginning any new diet, especially an extreme one, to rule out any possible risk owing to your previous medical history or present health condition. Sometimes, even a seemingly good thing might trigger a bad reaction when you have an underlying health condition.

Enough of the bad news. Now for the information you really want to hear. Green smoothies are gaining popularity as one of the healthiest things you can bring into your diet. The next chapter discusses the health benefits of green smoothies in detail.

Chapter 2: Extra-Galactic Benefits

"The food you eat can either be the safest most powerful form of medicine, or the slowest form of poison." Ann Wigmore

Green smoothies, when done properly, are so healthy that we haven't yet invented a word to describe just how good they are for your body. You'd have to travel all the way to The Andromeda Galaxy to find anything healthier. All right, perhaps I just made that up. But the following facts are incontrovertible:

Gets in your nine servings

Most people do not get the nine servings of fruits and vegetables per day that doctors recommend. Nine servings is about 4 ½ cups. When you make a smoothie and pulverize the food into a liquid, chances are good that you are going to consume quite a bit more of the vegetables and fruits than you would if you chewed them as solids. It just looks like less in liquid form. One smoothie has a good four fruit and vegetable servings.

Lowers the risk of heart disease

Green smoothies protect against heart disease on a number of levels. Many of the leafy greens are loaded with magnesium and other minerals that help lower cholesterol. Dietary fiber has also been associated with lowering bad cholesterol and increasing heart health as well. And losing weight helps out your heart most of all.

Lowers the risk of some cancers

Green smoothies are a rich source of antioxidants and anti-cancer phytochemicals which block the free radicals that can damage cells and even cause cancer.

Lowers the risk of type 2 diabetes

Increased consumption of magnesium and other minerals has been shown to lower the risk of type 2 diabetes. Losing weight lowers your risk as well.

Promotes weight loss

Changing to a diet rich in fruits and vegetables helps the body right itself in many aspects, including weight. The human body is a very efficient machine that has the ability to heal itself and also manage ideal weight when the food intake is the right kind. Processed and refined foods act against the body, disrupt its balance and result in illness. Green smoothies aid weight loss because they provide high energy and low caloric content while at the same time are extremely filling.

Hydrates the body

Green smoothies can help you maintain the right amount of water intake. As recommended by experts, an adult should drink about eight glasses of water daily. Most do not drink even half that number. If you count yourself among those who "forget" to drink water during the day, add two more glasses to the smoothie and you will be making up the quota without any trouble.

Maximizes nutritional intake

As mentioned in the last chapter, raw veggies have some advantages over cooked ones, in that cooking can destroy certain enzymes and vitamins like vitamin C. Many people rarely consume plain raw vegetables. We might dip them in dressing or hummus, or toss them in dressing, but snack on raw spinach? When you puree it with fruit, though, it becomes palatable without adding the extra calories, and you take full advantage of many of the vitamins and minerals.

Because the vegetables are pulverized, your body has a much easier time digesting the food and absorbing the nutrients, especially if you forget to listen to my grandmother and chew each mouthful twenty times before swallowing.

Even better when chewed

Speaking of chewing, even though green smoothies are liquid, it is a good practice to chew each mouthful a few times anyway. Huh? What? You may well ask. Digestion begins in the mouth, not in the gut. Some nutrients enter the body through the mouth. Give them a chance. Also, chewing activates certain enzymes, and it sets off one of those flashy light/sirens telling the stomach to prepare for incoming food. Finally, if you chew your smoothie, you will taste it, and you will be more likely to feel full when you are done.

Reduces time in the kitchen

It is much faster to prepare a smoothie than to cook, especially if you keep a tub of pre-washed spinach in the fridge and packages of fruit in the freezer. It is also pretty darn fast to consume, chewing included.

Prevents and cures constipation

Smoothies are different than juicing. Juicers spit out the pulp that is critical fiber that your body needs. When you juice, you have an alarming amount of messy waste. You need six times the fruits and vegetables just to fill a glass.

Generally, it is recommended that adults consume something around 25-30 grams of fiber every day. In reality, an adult in the USA typically consumes about 12 grams per day. Smoothies provide the much-needed fiber and hence, prevent and cure constipation.

Boots your inner and outer beauty

All those nutrients aren't just good for the inside. They are great for repairing cells and giving you glowing skin, shiny hair, and healthy nails.

Boosts energy levels

Dark leafy greens are great for boosting energy levels. In addition to the other vitamins and minerals, dark greens have chlorophyll, which helps distribute oxygen throughout the body. When you get more oxygen in your blood and brain (like when you exercise, ahem) you feel more alert.

Keeps you fuller longer

Chlorophyll has also been shown in studies to keep you feeling fuller longer. So does all that fiber, and any protein and fat that you add.

Promotes healthy teeth

Which is my way of reminding you to be sure to brush and floss your teeth after you drink a smoothie, for a couple of reasons. The first is that you will probably have berry seeds, and small spinach bits stuck between your teeth and in your gum line. Also the sugar from the broken down fruits and vegetables is going to stick to your teeth, and pretty soon you'll end up buying your dentist a new condo in Maui.

Broadens the palate

Some people find smoothies tough to adopt at first because of their strong taste. I compare it to sushi. The idea of raw fish was a little scary at first, but after a few California rolls, I graduated to rainbow rolls, and then I was hooked. Smoothies are the same way. Start off with more fruits, and gradually get more adventurous. Experiment with herbs and other flavors. Add peppers and ginger and even salsa for pep. Add cinnamon and anise and nutmeg for spunk. Some people will adapt faster than others, but at the end of eight days you will appreciate the flavors of vegetables more than ever.

Starts a great habit

Once you discover green smoothies, you will always have a healthy easy breakfast or lunch at your disposal.

Chapter 3: A Look at What Goes into a Smoothie

Do you carrot all for me?
My heart beets for you,
With your turnip nose
And your radish face,
You are a peach.
If we cantaloupe,
Lettuce marry;
Weed make a swell pear.

-Author Anonymous

The green smoothie is a blended mix of green leafy vegetables and other fruits, vegetables, and add-ins. They have shot to prime popularity owing to the many benefits they offer and their ability to help manage a number of serious diseases such as diabetes, cancer, heart problems, kidney problems, and liver problems.

Dr. Ann Wigmore invented the concept of green smoothies, and she's also the founder of Hippocrates Health Institute. She spent her life researching the connection between whole food and health. Ann's story is fascinating. A Lithuanian immigrant, she came to the United States in 1922 when she was a teenager. At some point, she developed gangrene in her leg. Rather than allow the doctors to amputate it, she began eating grass after observing that a sick cat has restored its health the same way. She credits the chlorophyll in the grass with saving her leg (and her life), and it inspired a lifelong passion. She was among the first to grow wheatgrass and drink it for health. She was also a vocal proponent of nut milks. Her hair remained its vibrant natural color well into her 80s, and she only required two hours of sleep a night. She said that she blended her food because she didn't want to "waste its energy, or mine."[1,2]

Thanks to Dr. Wigmore and other researchers who have studied how blending whole raw food can encourage the body to self-heal, there is an entire industry dedicated to green smoothies. But not all smoothies are created equal. Many of the chains that sell smoothies use sherbet for their bases and add sweeteners that have no business in a health and weight loss meal. Making your own is fast and easy, and it keeps the cost and quality under your control.

What Do You Put Into A Green Smoothie?

The best part about green smoothies is that they are very versatile, yet simple. You can literally put anything green you want in them. Normally it is made of 40:60 green leafy vegetables to fruits ratio. This is the recipe that will give you a most-palatable taste. As you get used to the taste the ratio can gradually up the greens to fruit ratio. The body doesn't need much sugar, even when it comes from fruit. The leafy vegetables are there for the nutrients, and everything else is in there to mask the taste of the greens and provide energy. My husband and I even make some without any fruits at all, kind of like a Bloody Mary mix without all the salt. Or vodka.

Once you get the idea of the what, how and why, you will want to start making your own green smoothies. In this chapter, I give you a basic recipe and include lots of variations at the end of the book to get you started, but don't stop there. When you find flavors you like, experiment and make it your own according to your taste and pleasure. Add other herbs and spices. Throw in what is fresh. Make

---

[1] http://www.rawfamily.com/dr-ann-wigmore

[2] http://rawfamily.com/news/2012/07/12-07-02.html

sure you use quality ingredients. Local produce tends to have more flavor and also more nutrients. Produce that has traveled halfway around the world was likely picked before it was ready and ripened on the way to the store. It is older, so the nutrients have started to degrade. Oddly enough, frozen produce, because it was picked and frozen immediately when ripe, tends to have maximum nutritional value. Feel free to experiment with frozen fruits and veggies in your creations. In fact, the more variety you experiment with, the better green smoothies you'll make. It takes experience to get just the right taste, texture and health benefits in a green glass.

Just remember that smoothies are best drank fresh. The nutrients start to degrade the moment you chop the foods up. If you do make a big batch, you can store it up to 48 hours in the refrigerator. If you refrigerate, shake the container well before you drink the smoothie and have it as soon as you bring out from the fridge. Do not allow it to warm up.

The ingredients that make a smoothie can be classified in the following categories: bases, leafy greens, fruits, fillers, spices, and superfoods. Please note that the lists you find are not all inclusive; rather they are indicative of what you could use to make excellent green smoothies. At the end of this book, you will find recipes that you can try out as they are or modify to suit your taste and the availability of local foods.

Perfect Green Smoothie: The Simplest Foolproof Formula

The basic green smooth recipe is as follows. It makes for two 16 oz. servings.

+ Leafy greens – 2 cups
+ Ripe fruit – 3 cups
+ Liquid base – 2 cups

Meal Replacement Green Smoothie

To make a smoothie filling enough to replace an entire meal, add superfoods, protein and fillers to the basic recipe.

+ Smoothie liquid – 2 cups
+ Fruit/ salad vegetables – 2 cups
+ Mild green leafy vegetables – 2 cups
+ Nuts/ seeds – ¼ cup or nut butter/ seed butter – 2 Tbsp.
+ Any one of the fillers listed below

You might need to drink half, and then wait thirty minutes to an hour and drink the other half.

Base (Liquid) Of the Smoothie

The "*base*" is the term used for the "*liquid*" added to the smoothie to make it drinkable. The normal measure is to use 2 cups of the base liquid. The best base is water. Here are my thoughts on the many bases I see listed in recipes

Water – Water is added so that the smoothie is the right consistency for drinking, and so your blender doesn't self-destruct. If you think you are not drinking enough water, add 1-2 cups more when you are making the smoothie, and get hydrated while you are getting your green goodness on.

Coconut Water – Coconut water is the clear liquid from the center of young, green coconuts. It has about 44 calories per cup. People are calling it the new sports drink because it is sweet and high in potassium and other electrolytes. If you use it, make sure to choose coconut water that doesn't have added fruit juice or sweeteners.

Coconut Milk – Coconut milk is made by extracting liquid from the meat of a coconut. Many people use it instead of milk and cream in paleo recipes, and it is definitely rich and yummy. I see a lot of smoothie recipes that use coconut milk because it makes them taste like a milkshake. Consider, though, that one cup of coconut milk adds 544 calories and 56 grams of fat, most of which is saturated fat. Compare that to a cup of heavy cream, which has 414 calories and 44 grams of fat, a little more than half of which is saturated. Coconut milk does have some micronutrients, like a little magnesium and potassium, but not as much as the green veggies. If you are trying to lose weight, I'd use coconut milk as sparingly as you would cream, at times when you are going to use the energy, like before a workout.

Fresh fruit juice – Fruit juice as a base adds nutrients and vitamins to the green smoothie, but not as much as using the whole fruit. It also adds sugar, typically about 24 grams per cup, and 113 calories. That is an entire day's RDA of sugar for most women. You should not use juice exclusively for the base if you are worried about the sugar content and weight loss. I stick with water and add cut up fruits for maximum nutritional benefit. If you do add juice, only add a little, and make sure it doesn't contain added sweeteners (even and especially artificial ones).

Nut milk (cashew, hemp, almond, etc.) – Nut milk is made by grinding nuts into a paste and then mixing in a lot of water. Nut milk adds a rich flavor, creaminess and a modest amount of calories if you chose the unsweetened brands. For example, a cup of almond milk had 40 calories, no fat, 1 gram of protein, vitamin A, and calcium. This is popular with people who prefer their green smoothies rich and creamy and are trying to lose weight at the same time. Nut milk also works for those who are lactose intolerant. But, instead of rushing out and buying nut milk, you can achieve the same end result by grinding up a tablespoon or two of nuts and then adding water to your smoothie.

Soy Milk – Soy milk is made by soaking soybeans in water and then grinding the mixture, sort of like a one ingredient smoothie. Soy milk has about 131 calories per cup, 4.2 grams of mostly unsaturated fat, 8 grams of protein, and quite a lot of magnesium, as well as calcium, iron, and potassium. It has some fiber, but the carbs are mostly sugar. Soy milk is great for meal replacement smoothies because the protein and fat help you to stay full longer, and it has lots of nutrients. It has a strong, some might say *acquired* taste.

Rice Milk – Rice milk, as you may have guessed, is made by soaking rice in water and blending it. It has a milder flavor than soy milk and is naturally sweet. Sometimes it is flavored with vanilla. With 120 calories per cup and 2 grams of unsaturated fat, it has a little calcium, no protein and not much else to benefit your body.

Skim Milk – Skim milk is made by removing the fat from whole milk via a centrifuge, and then adding back in milk solids and fortifying the product to make up for nutrients that went out with the fat. Skim milk has roughly 86 calories per cup, very little fat, 8 grams of protein, and half your daily calcium needs. It is also high in potassium, vitamin A, vitamin B12 and other nutrients, but also has lots of (natural) sugar.

2% Milk – 2% Milk has 122 calories per cup, 5 grams of fat (about half is saturated), 8 grams of protein, and lots of nutrients. It is made by removing all the fat and then adding some back in. Like skim milk, it is also high in sugar.

Whole Milk – Whole milk is somewhere between 3.5% - 4% fat and is the least processed form of cows' milk. It has 146 calories per cup, 8 grams of fat (a little over half is saturated), 8 g protein, lots of nutrients, and lots of sugar.

Artificially sweetened drinks – I see a lot of smoothie recipes that use artificially sweetened diet drinks as smoothie bases. Avoid these. They offer nothing in the way of nutrients, train your body to crave sweets, and can potentially contribute to serious health conditions. The diet industry is in the business of keeping the population fat.

Fruits

The best fruits to use for green smoothies are those which naturally sweeten your drink, mask the heavy taste of the greens, and provide the biggest nutritional spark. The sugar in fruits will give you quick energy, and the fiber, protein, and fat will give you the longer lasting kind. Mango and banana are popular because they add bright flavor and at the same time make the smoothie creamy and appetizing. I love adding apples, but some people don't because of the excess fiber. They also have a lot of sugar, so I only use small amounts. Other fruits to consider are avocado, berries, grapes, kiwi, papaya, peaches, pears and pineapple. Citrus fruit doesn't work very well unless you just add the juice. You can chop most fruit ahead of time and freeze them for cold smoothies. In fact, frozen berries top my list for both nutritional content and laziness factor. Remember that fruits are supposed to supplement, not replace the vegetables. For comparisons sake, here is the data on some of my favorites:

Apple – A large apple has 116 calories, no fat, .6 g protein, 5 g fiber, a fair amount of vitamin C and trace amounts of a variety of other essential nutrients.

Avocado – A whole avocado has 322 calories, 29 g of (mostly unsaturated) fat, 4 g protein, 13 g of fiber, and huge amounts of potassium, magnesium, vitamins C, E (great for skin), K, B-complex vitamins, and respectable amounts of most other essential vitamins and minerals. Because of the high fat concentration, avocados are great for early in the day when you are going to need energy.

Banana – A medium banana has 105 calories, .4 g of (mostly unsaturated) fat, 1.3 g of protein, 3 g fiber, and quite a lot of potassium, magnesium, manganese, B-complex vitamins, and Vitamin C, and trace amounts of other nutrients. Bananas are filling, have quick and slow energy, and make the smoothie thick and creamy.

Blackberries – Blackberries are my very favorite smoothie fruit. They have about 60 calories in a cup, 2 g of protein, 1 g of unsaturated fat, 8 g of fiber, and an appreciable amount of vitamins C & K and manganese, and trace amounts most other essential vitamins and minerals. They provide both immediate and long-lasting energy, fill you up, and you don't need to peel or segment them. You will, however, find seeds between your teeth.

Blueberries – Blueberries are a superfood. In one cup you get 85 calories, 1 g of protein, negligible fat, 4 g fiber, a ton of manganese, vitamins C & K, and a small amount of most other essential vitamins and minerals.

Cantaloupe – Half of a cantaloupe has 50 calories, no real fat, 1.5 g protein, 2 g fiber, more than your RDA of vitamins A & C, and minor amounts of most other essential vitamins and minerals.

Grape – Grapes have about 104 calories per cup, 1 g protein, 1 g fiber, and no appreciable fat. They are high in vitamins C & K and have detectable amounts of other nutrients. You don't need a lot of grapes to make your smoothie very sweet.

Kiwi – Kiwifruits pack a surprising amount of goodness inside their fuzzy little skins. A large kiwi has 56 calories, 1 g of protein, 3 g fiber, negligible fat, lots of vitamin K, and enough vitamin C to float an aircraft carrier. The downside is that they are a pain to peel.

Mango – Mangos are dense with nutrients. One mango has 135 calories, 1 g of unsaturated fat, 1 g of protein, 4 g of fiber, a day's worth of vitamin C and appreciable amounts of vitamins A, E, K, B-complex, potassium, and copper. They make a smoothie creamier, have both quick and long-lasting energy, and are filling. Their flaw is that they are tough to peel and weird to slice because of the odd stone.

Papaya – Papayas are another nutrient powerhouse fruit and one of my favorites. A medium papaya has 119 calories, negligible fat, 2 g protein, 5 g fiber, 3xs your RDA of vitamin C, and more than half of your daily A. They have respectable amounts of vitamins E, K, B-complex, and potassium, and trace amounts of others. They are an excellent choice to keep you full longer.

Peach – A large peach has a 68 calories, negligible fat, 1.6 g protein, 3 g fiber, and modest amounts of potassium, A & C. Peel them or leave the skin on, your choice.

Pear – A large pear has 133 calories, negligible fat, 1 g protein, 7 g of fiber, modest amounts of vitamins C & K, and a smattering of other vitamins and minerals.

Pineapple – If you choose canned pineapple, be careful about added sugar. A cup of fresh pineapple has 82 calories, 1 g protein, negligible fat, 2 g fiber, more than you need of C, 76% RDA of manganese, and trace amounts of other essential vitamins and minerals. Fresh pineapple is so tasty, and such a pain to cut. Frozen pineapple chunks work great for smoothies.

Raspberries – Raspberries are a spectacular fruit because they have about 64 calories in a cup, 1 g of unsaturated fat, 1.5 g of protein, and 8 g of fiber, so they are going to fill you up. They have half your daily C, respectable amounts of vitamin K and manganese, and traces of many other essential nutrients.

Watermelon – is sweet and watery, but won't give you much energy. One cup has 46 calories, no fat, 1 g fiber, 1 g protein, 20% RDA of C and A, and not much else.

Green Leafy Vegetables

Beet Greens - These greens are similar to spinach and chard, and you can use the beetroot too! Beet greens have about 40 calories per cup, 4 g each of protein and fiber, no fat, more than a day's requirement of vitamins A & K, and are have more than 20% of your RDA of vitamin C, riboflavin, magnesium, potassium, and manganese, and have more than 10% of vitamin E, thiamin, calcium, iron, B6, sodium, and copper.

Bok Choy - Also known as the Chinese cabbage, it has a slightly bitter taste but it can be easily overpowered by any sweet fruit you use. One cup has 20 calories, 3 g protein, 2 g fiber, no fat, excess vitamin A, more than 70% RDA of vitamins C & K, and more than

10% RDA of vitamin B6, folate, calcium, iron, potassium, and manganese.

Collard Greens - Collard greens have 49 calories per cup, 4 g protein, 5 g fiber, 1 g unsaturated fat, and crazy over-the-top amounts of vitamins A & K. They have half your vitamin C, 40% plus of manganese and folate, 20% plus of calcium, and at least 10% of riboflavin, B6, iron, and magnesium.

Dandelion Greens - An excellent detox agent, dandelion greens are often used for liver, gallbladder cleansing and promotion of kidney function. My grandmother swore by them for people experiencing painful kidney stones. One cup has 25 calories, no fat, 1 g protein, 2 g fiber, over-the-top vitamin A & K, 30% RDA of vitamin C, and 10% RDA of calcium and vitamin E.

Green And Red Leaf Lettuce - Green and red leaf lettuces are light in flavor and inexpensive. One cup of lettuce has 8 calories, .6 g of protein, 1 g of fiber, more than half your RDA of vitamins A & K, and more than 10% RDA of vitamin C & folate.

Kale - Kale is another superfood. One cup of kale has 33 calories, 2 g protein, 1 g fiber, and more than 100 RDA of vitamins A, C, & K, and 36% of your RDA of manganese, and 10% of RDA of copper, calcium, and potassium.

Mustard Greens – One cup of mustard greens has 21 calories, 3 g of protein, 3 g of fiber, no fat, and crazy amounts of vitamins A & K. They have half your C, a quarter of your folate, and 10% plus of calcium and manganese. These greens have a spicy flavor, so use them in small amounts to boost lettuce or spinach.

Parsley – Parsley has 22 calories per cup, 2 g of protein and two of fiber. It has ridiculous amounts of vitamins A, C, & K, more than 20% of your RDA of iron and folate and adding a little can enhance your smoothie's flavor.

Spinach - Spinach is the most common ingredient used for green smoothie because it is abundantly available, has a mild taste and lots of nutrients. One cup has seven calories, a g of protein, 1 g of fiber, and no fat. It has more than you need of vitamin K, half of your vitamin A, and more than 10% of your RDA for vitamin C, folate, and manganese. I like to get the big containers of pre-washed baby spinach for super-fast smoothies.

Swiss chard – A great alternative to spinach. It has seven calories per cup, .6 g of protein, and 1 g of fiber. It has 300% of your daily vitamin K, 44% of vitamin A, and 18% of vitamin C. Be aware that Chard is highly perishable; it should be consumed within 2-3 days maximum.

Turnip Greens – Turnip greens are a hot favorite for green smoothies, and one of the most overlooked leafy greens out there. Turnip green are similar in taste and texture to spinach, kale and collard greens. One cup has 29 calories, 2 g of protein and 5 of fiber. A serving has twice your daily A, six times your vitamin K requirements, 66% of your C, 42% of folate, and better than 10% of your RDA for vitamin E, B6, calcium, copper, and manganese.

Fillers

Fillers thicken the green smoothie and make it creamier. Some examples of foods that add volume and richness are avocado, buckwheat, butternut, oats, quinoa, squash, sweet potato and yogurt. I throw leftover baked sweet potatoes and squash into smoothies. The other fillers you can add raw.

Dairy Products

Yogurt – Add 1 cup of whole yogurt for 149 calories, 9 g of protein, and 8 g of (mostly saturated) fat. Be careful about added natural and artificial sweeteners.

Cottage cheese – 1 cup has 163 calories, 28 g of protein, and 2 g of fat.

Raw eggs – 1 egg has 78 calories, 6 g of protein, and 5 g of (mostly unsaturated) fat. Eggs are huge sources of vitamin B12, a critical vitamin that many vegetarians are deficient in. They are also a great source of other B-complex vitamins and iron. If raw eggs freak you out, poach or boil them first before adding to your smoothie.

Good Carbs

Sweet potato – 1 cup, baked or steamed, has 114 calories, 2 g protein, very little fat, and 4 g fiber. Sweet potatoes have better than 10% of your RDA of vitamins A, C, thiamin, riboflavin, niacin, B6, magnesium, phosphorus, potassium, copper, and manganese.

Squash – 1 cup, baked or steamed has 82 calories, 2 g protein, and little fat or fiber. Squash has better than 10% of your RDA of vitamins A, C, E, niacin, B6, folate, magnesium, potassium, and manganese.

Pumpkin – 1 cup of cooked pumpkin has 49 calories, no fat, 2 g protein, 2 g of fiber, tons of vitamin A, and more than 10% of your RDA of vitamins C, E, riboflavin, potassium, copper, and manganese.

Grains

Oats – 1/2 cup; soak them overnight in the liquid meant for the smoothie to make it creamy, or just add with extra water for texture. One ½ c (will be roughly 1 cup after it is soaked) has 300 calories, 5.5 g (mostly unsaturated) fat, 13 g protein, and 8.54 g fiber. Fortified oats have a ridiculous amount of micronutrients as well: all of the B complex vitamins except B12, and better than 20% of your daily iron, magnesium, phosphorus, zinc, and copper. Oats are a great addition if you are going to need a lot of energy.

Quinoa – 1/3 cup; soak them overnight in the liquid meant for the smoothie, and they will expand to roughly 1 cup. Or add with extra water for texture. One serving will have 222 calories, 4 g unsaturated fat, 8 g protein, 5 g fiber, B-complex vitamins, and more than 10% of your RDA of iron, magnesium, phosphorus, zinc copper, and manganese.

Buckwheat – 1/3 cup; rinse every 2 hours about four times, then add to the blender, or add with extra water. Buckwheat has about 200 calories, 2 g fat, 8 g protein, 6 g fiber. Fortified buckwheat is heavy on B complex vitamins and various minerals.

Nuts

Nuts – Grind up 1 oz. with your smoothie, and you'll add between 160-185 calories, 2-6 g of protein, 1-3 g of fiber, and 12-21 g of fat. Macadamia nuts have the least to offer you nutritionally. Almonds, cashews, pistachios, and peanuts (even though they aren't a nut) pack the biggest bang.

Nut butter – 2 tbsp. of nut butter is slightly heavier in calories and fat than plain nuts because of added oil, but otherwise, if you choose brands without added sugar, nut butter is nutritionally similar to plain nuts.

Seeds

Seeds – Grind up an ounce to give your smoothie some texture, or soak them overnight. Chia seeds are popular, but you can also add pumpkin seeds, sesame seeds, sunflower seeds, flax seeds, squash seeds, or whatever strikes your fancy. Seeds will add calories, protein, fat, and fiber, and some offer other mineral benefits.

Seed butter – 2 tbsp. of seed butter will give you a few more calories but otherwise similar nutritional content to the seeds, and it will be smoother.

Spices, Essential Oils, and Flavoring Herbs

These herbs are excellent additions in terms of nutrients and special attributes. However, when these are added to the green smoothies, this is done more to add flavor than for the nutrients' value. This is an indicative list; you could use any other spices/herbs that you find appetizing.

Basil – I love basil with lemon zest.

Cilantro – You love it, or you hate it. It is great with avocado, and smoothies that aren't sweet.

Cinnamon – Great with smoother smoothies, like with pumpkin and banana.

Cloves – My mother chews cloves as breath mints. Cloves are strong, so a little goes a long way.

Ginger – Peel the root and grind it with the veggies for some spice. It is great with both sweet and not-sweet smoothies.

Jalapeno – Grind it with the veggies for some spice. I like the combination with sweet, too.

Lemon, lime, and orange zest –Add a citrusy flavor.

Mint – You just need a few sprigs to flavor the whole smoothie. Combine it with pineapple or any type of berries.

Parsley – Parsley leaves lend a distinct flavor to the smoothie.

Vanilla extract – Great with sweet smoothies and with coconut water. It goes very well with cacao powder and berries.

Sweeteners

I see a lot of "green smoothie" recipes that include all kinds of sweeteners, from syrups, to honey, to molasses, to sherbet, to Crystal Light. Um, no. No, no, no, no, no, and no. For a lot of reasons.

The first is that if you are drinking green smoothies for weight loss and health, then don't add extra, empty calories. If you are adding fruit, or even vegetables like carrots and beets, you get nutrients along with the natural sugar. You can make them sweet enough with fruits and vegetables. Give it a chance.

The second is that when you stop sweetening things, you start to appreciate the other flavors. Fruits taste sweeter, other flavors taste richer. Give yourself some time to adjust, and fruit will magically start tasting completely different to you.

The third is that artificial sweeteners, fake sugars if you will, are a huge contributing factor to weight gain in the first place. When the body eats something sweet, it expects to get some energy along with it. When you consume no-calorie sweeteners, your appetite increases, and there is no corresponding feeling of satiation like that you get when you consume natural sugars. Add to that that so many artificial sweeteners are linked to some pretty scary health conditions, and you should avoid them like clichés.

Oils

I've also heard of people adding salad dressing to smoothies. Smoothies are not salads. Most bottled salad dressings use harmful oils and additives like sugar. The body does require some fat, as fat provides energy, helps your body absorb certain vitamins and minerals, and some types can even lower blood pressure and cholesterol. Only 20-35% of your calories should be from fat, and you should already be getting plenty from your fruits, and even more if you add avocado, nuts, eggs, dairy, or seeds to your smoothie. If you feel you need to add more fat, though, you can add a tbsp. of extra virgin olive oil or coconut oil.

Superfoods (add any 1 or 2)

The power of green smoothies is derived from the green vegetables and fresh fruits, and they are complete as is. However, some people add 1-2 superfoods to the mix to increase its potency. Some of these items have huge cult followings, and any outrageous claims should be analyzed critically. Still, try some of them out and see what you think. Experimenting can be fun, and you just never know.

Bee Superfoods

Bee pollen has almost seven times the amount of protein beef has. It is purported to help protect against allergies – particularly sinusitis and hay fever – but a top allergist I consulted said that was rubbish. He also warned that it could dramatically increase your allergic reaction, so be very careful, especially if your allergies are severe. Bee pollen is not safe for pregnant or breastfeeding women.

Propolis is a little-known substance that coats the walls of bee hives. Propolis has been shown to help strengthen the immune system and fight off viruses, bacteria, and fungi. It is not safe for pregnant women, and can be deadly to people who are allergic to bees or bee stings.

Royal jelly is a substance that is secreted by worker bees from a gland in the head. This is produced exclusively for feeding the Queen Bee. This is a rich source of Vitamin B5, which is a key compound for the health of hair, skin and fighting stress and stress-related insomnia. It might help lower blood pressure. Studies have shown it can help women with menopause-related symptoms. There are lots of other claims about royal jelly that have not been scientifically proven, but haven't been disproven either. Don't take it if you are allergic to bees or are pregnant.

Fruit, Nut, & Root Superfoods

Acai - The acai berries are a rich source of antioxidants, even more than blueberries, raspberries, and blackberries. Like their other berry cousins, acai berries are a great fruit for weight loss because they pack protein, fat, and fiber.

Coconut - In previous sections, we looked at adding coconut water, which is rich in antioxidants, and coconut milk, which has lots of saturated fats. Shredded, unsweetened coconut is mostly fat as well and has almost nothing in the way of micronutrients. Avoid coconut for weight loss.

Goji berries are exceptionally rich in vitamin C. These berries contain 500 times more Vitamin C per ounce than oranges. They also contain vitamins E, B6, B2, B1 and A, 18 essential amino acids and as many as 21 trace minerals. Goji berries are prized for their purported ability to reverse aging process and boost the immune system. Preliminary studies have shown that they promote a sense of calm and help with weight loss.

Maca is a root that indigenous Peruvians eat as a main staple because it is one of the few things that grows high in the Andes. Recently, it has gotten a reputation for increasing the libido, sort of a natural Viagra. It is also prized as a food that increases energy and promotes clear thinking. These claims have not been proven, but it is high in many essential minerals. It is supposed to have a very strong (unpleasant) taste.

Raw cacao is from the same plant that gives us chocolate, but is decidedly less tasty. It has enormous amounts of antioxidants and magnesium. Try it with some vanilla.

Ginseng is a tuber that has been used for thousands of years in Eastern medicine. Studies of ginseng in the West have shown it can boost the immune system, lower blood sugar, and (mildly) increase concentration. It is also being researched for a number of other benefits, like treating cancer, heart disease, and fatigue, and while the jury is still out, it has exciting potential. Talk to your doctor before taking ginseng because it can react with other medications.

Green Superfoods

Wheatgrass is the grass that sprouts from wheat seeds. The grass does not contain gluten. As a grass, it is difficult to digest, so people usually extract just the juice. Wheatgrass is extremely high in chlorophyll, vitamins A, C, E, K, and all of the B-Complex vitamins *except folate and B12*. It is also huge in the minerals iron, zinc, copper, and manganese. It has an obsessive following that claims it can cure cancer and AIDS and prevent gray hair, but, as of this printing, there is no actual evidence. Studies *have* shown it can help with chemotherapy side effects and also help with ulcerative colitis symptoms. It might also help ease arthritis and gout, and there is some evidence it helps with some bacterial infections. Wheatgrass also has some protein and fiber. It tastes the sweetest when it is youngest.

Barley grass has similar nutritional content to wheatgrass and a similar cult following. It is the grass sprouted from barley seeds, as opposed to wheat seeds. People who love it use it to treat everything under the sun. There is no evidence that barley grass is a miracle drug, but it is uncontrovertibly rich in vitamins and minerals. Many people like the taste of barley grass better than wheat grass.

Chlorella is a fresh water algae and known as a superfood because it has a lot of protein, fat, carbohydrates, fiber, vitamins, and minerals. There are claims that it helps with gastrointestinal issues and can help prevent cancer, but they have not been well-researched. Avoid wild algae because it could be contaminated by bacteria. Only consume algae grown in controlled environments.

Spirulina is a blue-green Algae that is rich in protein. Research in underway to see if it can help the immune system and viral infections. Again, avoid wild algae because it could be contaminated by bacteria. Only consume algae grown in controlled environments.

Wild blue-green algae has a checkered reputation. Depending on what source you read, it is either the world's most perfect food or a giant scam. It is a rich source of chlorophyll, protein, iron, and some of the B-complex vitamins. Again, be careful about possibly contaminated algae, and don't take this if you are pregnant, breastfeeding, and don't feed it to children.

Seaweed - Most people first experience seaweed wrapped around a piece of sushi, or in a salad. Seaweed is low in fat and calories but rich in protein, vitamins, and minerals and has been praised for helping to lower blood pressure. My kids eat dried seaweed as a crunchy snack, like kale chips, and it makes just as big a mess in the hands of a six-year-old as a packet of potato chips. Blended in a smoothie, seaweed can boost your nutrients, and the fruit can mask the fishy flavor if you're not a fan.

Herb Superfoods

Stinging Nettle is a wild green/weed that has prickly hairs on the stems and undersides of the leaves. The ancient Greeks revered it as a laxative, and throughout the centuries, people have used it to help fight inflammation and urinary tract issues. It is eaten as a green, or dried and steeped in tea. It is a good source of fiber, calcium, vitamin A, and magnesium.

Aloe Vera has two parts which are used medicinally: the gel and the latex. My grandmother always kept aloe vera plants and would crack open a leaf and spread the gel on our skin to soothe burns, sunburns, and skin rashes. As a topical remedy, it has been studied exhaustively, and there is evidence that it increases circulation and kills bacteria. But the latex used to be used in laxatives and is now banned because it has been found to be unsafe. In high doses, it might actually cause cancer and kidney disease. Both aloe vera gel and aloe vera latex are being studied as remedies for a variety of conditions, and there is promising research. But be careful. Aloe vera gel is considered safe to take orally. Aloe vera latex is considered possibly unsafe and is "likely unsafe in high doses".[3]

Echinacea is a beautiful pink flower related to the daisy. Its leaves, flowers, and stems are dried and used as a tea, or juiced when fresh. There is evidence that Echinacea is effective in decreasing inflammation, stimulating the immune system, and attacking the yeast and other fungi. It is commonly used as a cold remedy, and it is possible that it might prevent infection as well. Wilder claims have not been substantiated.

Gingko Biloba - Leaves from the Gingko Biloba tree are used to make an extract that is another staple of Eastern medicine. There is strong evidence that Gingko Biloba increases blood flow to the brain and other areas. It has been used effectively to treat and slow the

---

[3] http://www.webmd.com/vitamins-supplements/ingredientmono-607-aloe.aspx?activeingredientid=607&activeingredientname=aloe

progression of memory problems, including symptoms of dementia, although it does not prevent dementia. It can help with clogged arteries, and also with symptoms of PMS, and it is being studied for effectiveness in other conditions. Check with your doctor about interactions with other drugs, and start with low doses.

Noni refers to compounds made from the leaves, roots, flowers, stems and bark of a certain kind of Evergreen tree. Medicines made with it are credited with curing everything from smallpox to cataracts to viruses on your computer. None of the claims have been medically recognized, but it is a rich source of phytonutrients, enzymes, minerals and vitamins.

Chapter 4: Green Smoothies Essentials

"Give me six hours to chop down a tree and I will spend the first four sharpening the ax." Commonly attributed to Abraham Lincoln

To ensure that you can make great green smoothies, you need appropriate tools as well as quality ingredients. We have talked about ingredients and their benefits in the earlier chapters. It is time we looked at the tools you need to make them.

The tools and other items described here can easily be bought online from Amazon.com as well as in scores of other online and offline markets. Before you buy, read reviews and compare prices to make sure you are getting both quality and value.

The Tools You Need

Blender

For the record, I have never tried to make a smoothie in a regular blender. I have pulverized onions in one, and it worked just fine. I asked the question of my reliable friend Google, and she had 241,000 different opinions on the subject. The consensus seems to be yeeeeeeeessssssssssswellmaybe. The caveats are: use lots of liquid, chop the pieces smaller yourself first, don't use ice, freeze the really stringy veggies like kale before you blend, and add the veggies last after you've blended everything else. Prepare smoothies in a regular blender at your own risk, and be gentle on the motor.

Just as I would recommend buying quality pots and pans, the right tool can make preparing your smoothies much, much easier. Some of the special blender manufacturers to consider are: Vitamix, Blendtec, NutriBullet, Ninja, and Oster.

For the record, if you are up for buying a piece of specialized equipment, I heartily recommend the NutriBullet, and they haven't paid me a dime. Pricewise it seems to be the middle of the road. I like it because it is easy to clean, everything but the base is dishwasher safe (and you don't need to clean that part), it works well, takes up very little room in the cupboard, and mine has lasted for years.

Pint-sized Mason Jars

Mason jars are hot favorites for smoothies, cocktails, and even coffee. They are beautiful, multi-functional and what is most important, reusable. Since they come with a wide mouth, they are easy to clean, too.

Ecojarz Lids

Ecojarz lids are mason jar lids with a hole for a straw, so you can drink your smoothie on the way to work without spilling it.

Dishwasher safe cutting board

No matter how great your blender is, you're apt to be doing a lot of cutting fruits and greens into chunks. Make sure you have a large cutting board that you can wash in the dishwasher that has a trench running around the edge to catch liquid.

Sharp knives and scissors

Your knives and kitchen shears are going to get a workout. Have them sharpened before you begin a smoothie diet.

Water Filter

We have great tap water where I live, but if you don't, a water filter can help your smoothies out quite a bit.

Straws

Invest in a large packet of big milkshake straws. They are disposable, but you can usually get away with washing them in the dishwasher a few times.

10 Tips and Tricks

It takes time to master the art of making green smoothies and just like anything else, a few tips and tricks are helpful whether you are a newbie or a veteran.

Training To Like Green Smoothies

Green smoothies take some getting used to. You need to train your taste buds to like them. Start with 40:60 greens to fruits ratio. If you do not like it, reduce the greens to 20 percent and increase it as your acceptance level builds up.

Chop first

Make your blender's job easier, and your smoothies smoother by chopping fruits and veggies first (make sure to save and add all the liquid).

Blend in Stages

To keep your smoothies from becoming chunkies, blend in stages. Put in your liquid base, then blend in the rest of ingredients, one group at a time – i.e. fruits, fillers, etc., with your greens last.

Freeze your fruit

You will find many recipes that call for ice. Instead, freeze the fruits you are planning to use after chopping them and use these cut and frozen fruits when you are making your smoothie. You can also freeze your greens too. Or, buy frozen fruits and veggies to begin with. As discussed in a previous chapter, frozen produce is picked at optimal times and frozen at its peak, so frozen produce can be higher in nutrients than the fresh. It is certainly faster.

The Best Sweetener

Use naturally sweet fruits such as pears, mangos, peaches, and bananas instead of adding additional sweeteners.

Work Up Gradually

Start with greens that do not directly assault your taste buds – like spinach. Spinach has a neutral taste, which means that no matter how much you put in, the smoothie will still taste like the fruit. You can use kale, too as it is extremely healthy and has a mild taste. Gradually add a little extra greens to your spinach and as you get used to the taste and work up to stronger tasting and more nutrient-packed greens like turnip greens.

Creamy smoothies

When starting out, people usually prefer a creamy texture to a watery one. Get this by using bananas, peaches, avocado, pears and papaya.

Repair kit

Sometimes, you'll end up with too strong a taste. To make it palatable use some natural sweetener/ flavor such as raw honey, vanilla extract or lemon juice. You may also add sweet fruits such as dates, pear, apple, grapes, peach and mango.

Plan ahead

Green smoothies take time to make; if you are not a morning person, try one of these shortcuts:

Make your smoothie in your free time and then store it in the refrigerator in an air-tight jar. Green smoothies can be refrigerated up to 48 hours. Before you drink a stored smoothie, shake it well.

Chop all the greens and fruits you like to use and store them in Ziploc bags or Tupperware. Mix what you need every morning to make a phenomenal green smoothie in less than 5 minutes.

Spice it up

Don't get stuck in a rut. Use spices and or herbs such as basil, mint, coriander, dill, lemon, ginger, jalapeno, cinnamon, etc. Not only they add a distinct flavor, but also add their own health benefits to the drink.

Conclusion

Green smoothies can make amazing additions to your daily nutrition and help you lose weight rapidly and stay healthy. These drinks come with remarkable properties and benefits, and can become a delicious lifetime habit.

Use these guidelines and start slowly. Give yourself time to adjust to the taste of green smoothies, and be prepared to overcome a little inertia in the beginning. You will feel healthier from the first drink, and you'll start seeing the benefits right away, even if it takes a little time before you really enjoy them.

Be adventurous and try out different ingredients and combinations until you find your own favorites. There are many sites which will give you wonderful recipes, but the best recipes will be those which you concoct according to your taste. Taken daily, you will find that you look younger, feel more energetic and are healthier than ever before. Welcome to the magic of green smoothies, which is rapidly converting people all over the world to a healthier lifestyle.

If you've found this book helpful, I'd appreciate it if you would take a minute or two to post a quick review. Your comments are the best way to help other readers determine if this book should be on their short list.

Have fun and stay healthy!

Cheers!

25 Luscious Green Smoothie Recipes to Get You Started

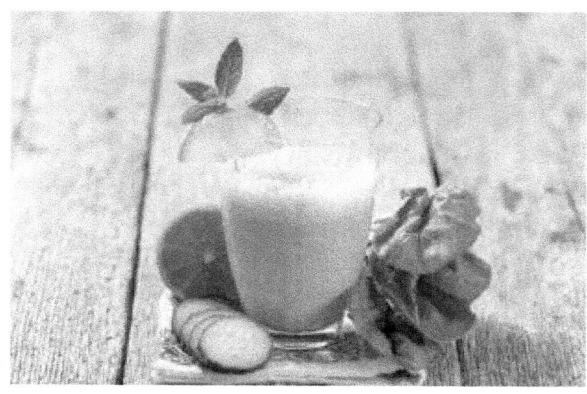

Green Smoothies Recipes Basic Formula

- Leafy greens – 2 cups
- Ripe fruit – 3 cups
- Liquid base – 2 cups
- Filler
- Spices

Blend in the order of base + fruit + filler + spices/ herbs/ superfoods + leafy greens

The RDA/ DV of Vitamins and other nutrients are calculated using the help of a free calculator on www.caloriecount.com. Use it for free, or any number of other apps, to measure the nutritional content of any meal you make.

Pumpkin Green Smoothie

Ingredients:
- 1 oz. raw or roasted (no salt) almonds
- 2 c water
- ½ apple, cored
- 1 cup cooked or canned pumpkin
- ½ tsp ground cinnamon
- 2 c baby spinach

Directions:
1. Soak the almonds overnight in the liquid base if you wish.
2. Grind the almonds in a blender or grinder.
3. Add the liquid base if you did not soak the almonds in it.
4. Add the apple, cinnamon powder, and pumpkin.
5. Add the baby spinach.
6. Blend at the highest speed for 30-45 seconds.

Nutrition Facts	
Serving Size 1 Serving	
% Based on 2000 Calorie Diet	
Per Serving	% Daily Value
Calories 275	13.75%
Calories from Fat 133	
Total Fat 14.8g	23%
Saturated Fat 1.2g	6%
Cholesterol 0mg	0%
Sodium 65mg	3%
Potassium 1210mg	35%
Carbohydrates 33.2g	11%
Dietary Fiber 10.0g	40%
Sugars 13.4g	
Protein 9.7g	
Vitamin A 357%	Vitamin C 59%
Calcium 19%	Iron 25%

This smoothie is low in saturated fat and sodium, and has no cholesterol. It is high in dietary fiber, manganese, magnesium, potassium, riboflavin, vitamin A, vitamin B6, vitamin C, & vitamin E.

Strawberry Mango Smoothie

Ingredients:
- 2 c water
- ½ c frozen mango
- 8 strawberries
- 2 c dandelion greens
- Flax seeds – 1 tbsp.
- Raw protein powder – 1 scoop (optional)

Directions:
1. Add the liquid base in the blender first.
2. Add the mango and strawberry.
3. Add the dandelion greens and flax seeds.
4. Add the protein powder.
5. Blend at the highest speed for 30-45 seconds.

Nutrition Facts

Serving Size 1 Serving
% Based on 2000 Calorie Diet

Per Serving	% Daily Value
Calories 247	12.35%
Calories from Fat 41	
Total Fat 4.5g	7%
Saturated Fat 1.0g	5%
Cholesterol 32mg	11%
Sodium 130mg	5%
Potassium 889mg	25%
Carbohydrates 38.4g	13%
Dietary Fiber 9.5g	38%
Sugars 21.0g	
Protein 9.7g	
Vitamin A 239%	Vitamin C 205%
Calcium 30%	Iron 35%

This smoothie is low in saturated fat and sodium, and is high in calcium, dietary fiber, iron, manganese, potassium, thiamin, vitamin A, vitamin B6, and vitamin C.

Sunflower Carrot Smoothie

Ingredients:
+ 2 tbsp. sunflower butter or 1 oz. sunflower seeds
+ 2 c water
+ 2 medium carrots cut into pieces
+ 2 celery stalks cut and frozen
+ 2 cups baby spinach (or any green leafy veggie)

Directions:
1. Add the sunflower butter or seeds.
2. Add the liquid base.
3. Add the carrot and celery.
4. Add the baby spinach.
5. Blend at the highest speed for 30-45 seconds.

Nutrition Facts

Serving Size 1 Serving
% Based on 2000 Calorie Diet

Per Serving	% Daily Value
Calories 262	13.1%
Calories from Fat 141	
Total Fat 15.6g	24%
Saturated Fat 1.7g	8%
Cholesterol 0mg	0%
Sodium 362mg	15%
Potassium 956mg	27%
Carbohydrates 25.3g	8%
Dietary Fiber 5.6g	22%
Sugars 7.3g	
Protein 9.6g	
Vitamin A 528%	Vitamin C 46%
Calcium 17%	Iron 20%

This smoothie has no cholesterol, and is high in manganese, magnesium phosphorus, potassium, vitamin A, vitamin B6, and vitamin C.

Grapes Green Smoothie

Ingredients:
+ 1 c water
+ 1/2 c red grapes
+ 1 c chopped frozen banana
+ 1 handful Italian parsley
+ 2 c baby spinach
+ ½ scoop protein powder

Instructions:
1. Add the liquid base in the blender first.
2. Add the banana.
3. Add the red grapes and Italian parsley.
4. Add the baby spinach.
5. Blend at the highest speed for 30-45 seconds.

Nutrition Facts

Serving Size 1 Serving
% Based on 2000 Calorie Diet

Per Serving	% Daily Value
Calories 282	14.1%
Calories from Fat 22	
Total Fat 2.4g	4%
Saturated Fat .8g	4%
Cholesterol 32mg	11%
Sodium 119mg	5%
Potassium 1445mg	41%
Carbohydrates 55.6g	19%
Dietary Fiber 7.9g	32%
Sugars 31.6g	
Protein 16.7g	
Vitamin A 217%	Vitamin C 188%
Calcium 22%	Iron 35%

This smoothie is low in saturated fat and sodium, high in dietary fiber, iron, manganese, magnesium, potassium, vitamin A, vitamin B6, and high vitamin C.

Berry Smoothie

Ingredients:
- 2 c water
- 2 tbsp. hazelnut butter
- 1/2 c strawberry
- 2 c frozen berries
- 2 c kale
- 2 c water

Instructions:
1. Add the liquid base in the blender first.
2. Add the berries and hazelnut butter.
3. Add the kale.
4. Blend at the highest speed for 30-45 seconds.

Nutrition Facts

Serving Size 1 Serving
% Based on 2000 Calorie Diet

Per Serving	% Daily Value
Calories 308	15.4%
Calories from Fat 62	
Total Fat 6.9g	11%
Saturated Fat .4g	2%
Cholesterol 0mg	0%
Sodium 73mg	3%
Potassium 1197mg	34%
Carbohydrates 55.1g	18%
Dietary Fiber 14.4g	58%
Sugars 23.9g	
Protein 7.9g	
Vitamin A 412%	Vitamin C 439%
Calcium 26%	Iron 24%

This smoothie is low in saturated fat and sodium, and it has no cholesterol. It is high in dietary fiber, manganese, potassium, vitamin A, and vitamin C.

Superfood Goji Berry Green Smoothie

Ingredients:
- 2 c water
- 1 kiwi fruit
- 1 banana cut up and frozen
- 4 tbsp. goji berries
- 1 tbsp. cacao powder
- 1/2 c Italian parsley
- 1 ½ c baby spinach

Instructions:
1. Add the liquid base in the blender first.
2. Add the kiwi fruit, banana, goji berry, cacao powder.
3. Add the Italian parsley.
4. Add the baby spinach.
5. Blend at the highest speed for 30-45 seconds.

Nutrition Facts

Serving Size 1 Serving
% Based on 2000 Calorie Diet

Per Serving	% Daily Value
Calories 294	14.7%
Calories from Fat 62	
Total Fat 3.6g	6%
Saturated Fat .8g	4%
Cholesterol 0mg	0%
Sodium 142mg	6%
Potassium 998mg	29%
Carbohydrates 71.6g	24%
Dietary Fiber 12.5g	50%
Sugars 25.7g	
Protein 8.9g	
Vitamin A 280%	Vitamin C 235%
Calcium 18%	Iron 21%

This green smoothie is low in saturated fat and sodium, and has no cholesterol. It is high in dietary fiber, vitamin A, and vitamin C.

Superfood Pear Green Smoothie

Ingredients:
+ 1 c soy milk
+ 1 c water
+ 1 pear sliced
+ 2 tsp chia seeds soaked for15-30 minutes in water
+ 1 in. ginger root peeled and chopped roughly
+ 1 large carrot
+ 2 c Swiss chard

Instruction:
1. Add the liquid base in the blender first.
2. Add the pear, fresh ginger, and Chia seeds.
3. Add the carrot, and Swiss chard.
4. Blend at the highest speed for 30-45 seconds.

Nutrition Facts

Serving Size 1 Serving
% Based on 2000 Calorie Diet

Per Serving	% Daily Value
Calories 275	13.8%
Calories from Fat 57	
Total Fat 6.3g	10%
Saturated Fat .6g	3%
Cholesterol 0mg	0%
Sodium 344mg	14%
Potassium 992mg	28%
Carbohydrates 48.3g	16%
Dietary Fiber 10.4g	42%
Sugars 27.7g	
Protein 11.4g	
Vitamin A 329%	Vitamin C 53%
Calcium 19%	Iron 21%

This green smoothie is low in saturated fat and has no cholesterol. It is high in dietary fiber, manganese, magnesium, potassium, vitamin A, and vitamin C.

Antioxidant Kale Green Smoothie

Ingredients:
- 2 c water
- 1 c banana frozen in chunks
- 1 c frozen or fresh blueberries
- 2 tbsp. orange zest
- 2 tbsp. orange juice
- 2 c kale
- 1/2 c spinach

Instructions:
1. Add the liquid base in the blender first.
2. Add the banana.
3. Add the blueberries, orange zest, and orange juice.
4. Add the baby kale and spinach.
5. Blend at the highest speed for 30-45 seconds.

Nutrition Facts

Serving Size 1 Serving
% Based on 2000 Calorie Diet

Per Serving	% Daily Value
Calories 308	15.4%
Calories from Fat 10	
Total Fat 1.1g	2%
Saturated Fat .2g	1%
Cholesterol 0mg	0%
Sodium 61mg	3%
Potassium 1394mg	40%
Carbohydrates 75.5g	25%
Dietary Fiber 10.7g	43%
Sugars 35.4g	
Protein 7.1g	
Vitamin A 415%	Vitamin C 399%
Calcium 21%	Iron 28%

This green smoothie has no cholesterol and is very low in sodium and saturated fat. It is high in dietary fiber, manganese, potassium, vitamin A, vitamin B6, and vitamin C.

Heart Healthy Avocado Green Smoothie

Ingredients:
+ 2 c water
+ 1 tbsp. ground flax seeds
+ 2 c frozen berries
+ 1/2 c avocado
+ 2 c baby spinach

Instructions:
1. Add the liquid base in the blender first.
2. Add the berries and flax seeds.
3. Add the avocado.
4. Add the baby spinach.
5. Blend at the highest speed for 30-45 seconds.

Nutrition Facts

Serving Size 1 Serving
% Based on 2000 Calorie Diet

Per Serving	% Daily Value
Calories 360	18%
Calories from Fat 159	
Total Fat 17.7g	27%
Saturated Fat 3.3g	17%
Cholesterol 0mg	0%
Sodium 68mg	3%
Potassium 1110mg	32%
Carbohydrates 44.5g	15%
Dietary Fiber 18.1g	72%
Sugars 20.7g	
Protein 6.4g	
Vitamin A 115%	Vitamin C 140%
Calcium 12%	Iron 31%

This green smoothie has no cholesterol, and is low in sodium. It is high in dietary fiber, vitamin A, vitamin B6, and vitamin C.

Cucumber and Melon Green Smoothie

Ingredients:
+ 1 oz. almonds (no salt) raw or roasted
+ 2 c water
+ 1 c cantaloupe
+ ½ cucumber unpeeled
+ 1 tsp lime juice
+ 6-10 mint leaves
+ 2 c dandelion greens

Instructions:
1. Soak the almonds overnight, or not, if desired.
2. Grind the almonds and add the water.
3. Add the cantaloupe, cucumber and lime juice.
4. Add the dandelion greens and mint leaves.
5. Blend at the highest speed for 30-45 seconds.

Nutrition Facts

Serving Size 1 Serving
% Based on 2000 Calorie Diet

Per Serving	% Daily Value
Calories 289	14.5%
Calories from Fat 139	
Total Fat 15.4g	24%
Saturated Fat 1.4g	7%
Cholesterol 0mg	0%
Sodium 126mg	5%
Potassium 1287mg	37%
Carbohydrates 34.4g	11%
Dietary Fiber 9.5g	38%
Sugars 16.7g	
Protein 11.3g	
Vitamin A 332%	Vitamin C 167%
Calcium 33%	Iron 29%

This smoothie has no cholesterol and is low in sodium. It is high in calcium, dietary fiber, manganese, magnesium, potassium, riboflavin, vitamin A, and vitamin C.

Goji Berry and Cantaloupe Green Smoothie

Ingredients:
+ 2 c water
+ 1/3 c whole oats
+ 1 c cantaloupe frozen
+ 2 c baby kale
+ 4 tbsp. goji berries

Instructions:
1. Soak the oats overnight for a smoother texture, if desired.
2. Soak the goji berries in water for 10 minutes.
3. Add the cantaloupe.
4. Add the baby kale and goji berries.
5. Blend at the highest speed for 30-45 seconds.

Nutrition Facts

Serving Size 1 Serving
% Based on 2000 Calorie Diet

Per Serving	% Daily Value
Calories 304	15.2%
Calories from Fat 29	
Total Fat 3.2g	3%
Saturated Fat .4g	2%
Cholesterol 0mg	0%
Sodium 85mg	4%
Potassium 1173mg	34%
Carbohydrates 62.3g	21%
Dietary Fiber 8.3g	33%
Sugars 27.5g	
Protein 9.6g	
Vitamin A 520%	Vitamin C 387%
Calcium 21%	Iron 68%

This smoothie has no cholesterol and is very low in saturated fat and sodium. It is high in dietary fiber, iron, manganese, potassium, vitamin A, and vitamin C.

Apples and Cinnamon Green Smoothie

Ingredients:
- 1 cup of water
- 1 c plain yogurt
- 1 apple sliced
- 1 teaspoon cinnamon
- 2 c baby spinach

Instructions:
1. Add the liquid base in the blender first.
2. Add the yogurt.
3. Add the apple and cinnamon.
4. Add the baby spinach.
5. Blend at the highest speed for 30-45 seconds.

Nutrition Facts

Serving Size 1 Serving
% Based on 2000 Calorie Diet

Per Serving	% Daily Value
Calories 288	14.4%
Calories from Fat 32	
Total Fat 3.6g	6%
Saturated Fat 2.5g	13%
Cholesterol 15mg	5%
Sodium 224mg	9%
Potassium 1114mg	32%
Carbohydrates 46.4g	15%
Dietary Fiber 7.0g	28%
Sugars 36.5g	
Protein 16.3g	
Vitamin A 115%	Vitamin C 55%
Calcium 54%	Iron 16%

This green smoothie is low in cholesterol, and is high in calcium, manganese, phosphorus, potassium, riboflavin, vitamin A, vitamin B6, and vitamin C.

Celery and Broccoli Green Smoothie

Ingredients:
+ 1 c water
+ 1 c soymilk
+ 1 tangerine
+ ½ teaspoon grated ginger powder, or 1 in. fresh ginger peeled and chopped roughly
+ 4 celery stalks
+ 8 broccoli florets

Instructions:
1. Add the liquid base in the blender first.
2. Add the tangerine, celery, and grated ginger
3. Add the broccoli.
4. Blend at the highest speed for 30-45 seconds.

Nutrition Facts

Serving Size 1 Serving
% Based on 2000 Calorie Diet

Per Serving	% Daily Value
Calories 269	13.4%
Calories from Fat 43	
Total Fat 4.8g	7%
Saturated Fat 0.6g	3%
Cholesterol 0mg	0%
Sodium 229mg	10%
Potassium 1099mg	31%
Carbohydrates 47.9g	16%
Dietary Fiber 6.8g	27%
Sugars 34.4g	
Protein 12.7g	
Vitamin A 60%	Vitamin C 281%
Calcium 17%	Iron 17%

This green smoothie is low in saturated fat and has no cholesterol. It is high in manganese, magnesium, potassium, vitamin A, and vitamin C.

Blueberry Antioxidant Green Smoothie

Ingredients:
- 1 oz. raw or roasted almonds (no salt)
- 2 c water
- 1 c banana frozen and chopped
- ½ c fresh or blueberries
- 100 g frozen Acai puree
- ½ c pomegranate arils (seed pods)
- 2 c kale

Instructions:
1. Soak the almonds overnight in the liquid if desired.
2. Grind almonds in the blender and add the liquid.
3. Add the banana, blueberries, and acai puree.
4. Add the pomegranate seeds and the kale.
5. Blend at the highest speed for 30-45 seconds.

Nutrition Facts

Serving Size 1 Serving
% Based on 2000 Calorie Diet

Per Serving	% Daily Value
Calories 441	22%
Calories from Fat 139	
Total Fat 15.4g	24%
Saturated Fat 1.3g	7%
Cholesterol 0mg	0%
Sodium 62mg	3%
Potassium 1459mg	42%
Carbohydrates 65.3g	22%
Dietary Fiber 12.7g	51%
Sugars 26.7g	
Protein 12.7g	
Vitamin A 414%	Vitamin C 309%
Calcium 26%	Iron 26%

This green smoothie has no cholesterol and is low in saturated fat and sodium. It is high in dietary fiber, manganese, vitamin A, vitamin B6, and vitamin C.

Kiwi Banana Green Smoothie

Ingredients:
+ 1/3 c whole wheat
+ 2 c water
+ 2 kiwi fruit peeled and chopped
+ 1 banana, chopped, frozen
+ 2 c radish greens

Instructions:
1. Soak the wheat overnight in the liquid if desired.
2. Add the liquid and wheat to the blender.
3. Add the kiwi fruit and banana.
4. Add the radish greens.
5. Blend at the highest speed for 30-45 seconds.

Nutrition Facts

Serving Size 1 Serving
% Based on 2000 Calorie Diet

Per Serving	% Daily Value
Calories 431	21.5%
Calories from Fat 16	
Total Fat 1.8g	3%
Saturated Fat 0.2g	1%
Cholesterol 0mg	0%
Sodium 42mg	2%
Potassium 1457mg	42%
Carbohydrates 101.8g	34%
Dietary Fiber 18.4g	74%
Sugars 32.9g	
Protein 12.5g	
Vitamin A 63%	Vitamin C 316%
Calcium 27%	Iron 29%

This green smoothie has no cholesterol and is low in saturated fat and sodium. It is high in dietary fiber, manganese, selenium, vitamin A, and vitamin C.

Pineapple and Papaya Green Smoothie

Ingredients:
- 1 oz. walnuts raw or roasted (no salt)
- 2 c water
- 2 tbsp. coconut milk
- 1 c pineapple cubes frozen
- 1 c papaya cubes frozen
- 2 c baby spinach

Instructions:
1. If desired, soak the walnuts overnight in the liquid.
2. Grind the walnuts.
3. Add the water and the coconut milk.
4. Add the papaya and pineapple.
5. Add the baby spinach.
6. Blend at the highest speed for 30-45 seconds.

Nutrition Facts

Serving Size 1 Serving
% Based on 2000 Calorie Diet

Per Serving	% Daily Value
Calories 402	20.1%
Calories from Fat 222	
Total Fat 24.7g	38%
Saturated Fat 7.4g	37%
Cholesterol 0mg	0%
Sodium 74mg	3%
Potassium 1008mg	29%
Carbohydrates 44.0g	15%
Dietary Fiber 8.7g	35%
Sugars 29.1g	
Protein 10.8g	
Vitamin A 143%	Vitamin C 309%
Calcium 14%	Iron 21%

This green smoothie has no cholesterol and is low in sodium. It is high in manganese, magnesium, vitamin A, and vitamin C.

Strawberry and Lemon Green Smoothie

Ingredients:

+ 1 c water
+ 1 c soymilk
+ 1 banana frozen and chopped
+ 6 strawberries
+ ½ lemon peeled
+ ½ teaspoon lemon zest
+ 2 c turnip greens

Instructions:

1. Add the liquid base in the blender first.
2. Add the strawberries, banana, lemon and lemon zest.
3. Add the turnip greens.
4. Blend at the highest speed for 30-45 seconds.

Nutrition Facts

Serving Size 1 Serving
% Based on 2000 Calorie Diet

Per Serving	% Daily Value
Calories 296	14.8%
Calories from Fat 47	
Total Fat 5.2g	8%
Saturated Fat 0.7g	3%
Cholesterol 0mg	0%
Sodium 178mg	7%
Potassium 1153mg	33%
Carbohydrates 55.9g	19%
Dietary Fiber 9.6g	38%
Sugars 28.7g	
Protein 11.5g	
Vitamin A 257%	Vitamin C 200%
Calcium 30%	Iron 19%

This green smoothie has no cholesterol and is low in saturated fat. It is high in dietary fiber, manganese, magnesium, potassium, vitamin A, vitamin B6, and vitamin C.

Citrus Blackberry Kale Green Smoothie

Ingredients:
- 1 oz. pecans
- 2 c water
- 1 c frozen blackberries
- 1 orange peeled without seeds
- ½ lemon peeled without seeds
- 2 c kale

Instructions:
1. Soak the pecans in the liquid overnight, if desired.
2. Grind the pecans and add the liquid base if not soaked.
3. Add the frozen blackberries, orange, and lemon.
4. Add the kale.
5. Blend at the highest speed for 30-45 seconds.

Nutrition Facts

Serving Size 1 Serving
% Based on 2000 Calorie Diet

Per Serving	% Daily Value	
Calories 412	20.6%	
Calories from Fat 191		
Total Fat 21.2g	33%	
Saturated Fat 2.1g	11%	
Cholesterol 0mg	0%	
Sodium 74mg	3%	
Potassium 1346mg	38%	
Carbohydrates 53.5g	18%	
Dietary Fiber 17.1g	68%	
Sugars 25.2g		
Protein 10.8g		
Vitamin A 427%	Vitamin C 482%	
Calcium 33%	Iron 22%	

This green smoothie has no cholesterol and is low in sodium. It is high in dietary fiber, manganese, vitamin A, and vitamin C.

Pomegranate and Pear Green Smoothie

Ingredients:
+ 2 c water
+ ½ scoop raw protein powder
+ 1 c frozen blueberries
+ ½ tsp. maca powder
+ 2 tbsp. goji berries
+ 1 pear sliced
+ 2 tbsp. pomegranate seeds
+ 2 c dandelion greens

Instructions:
1. Add the liquid base in the blender first.
2. Add the blueberries, protein powder, maca, and goji berries.
3. Add the pear and pomegranate seeds.
4. Add the dandelion greens.
5. Blend at the highest speed for 30-45 seconds.

Nutrition Facts

Serving Size 1 Serving
% Based on 2000 Calorie Diet

Per Serving	% Daily Value
Calories 333	16.7%
Calories from Fat 22	
Total Fat 2.5g	4%
Saturated Fat 0.6g	3%
Cholesterol 31mg	10%
Sodium 128mg	5%
Potassium 880mg	25%
Carbohydrates 69.9g	23%
Dietary Fiber 14.0g	56%
Sugars 38.6g	
Protein 15.7g	
Vitamin A 225%	Vitamin C 121%
Calcium 29%	Iron 34%

This green smoothie is low in saturated fat and sodium. It is high in dietary fiber, iron, vitamin A, vitamin B6, and vitamin C.

Fig and Pear Green Smoothie

Ingredients:

+ 2 c water
+ 1 oz. almonds raw or roasted (no salt)
+ ½ c ice
+ 1 pear sliced
+ ½ tsp. vanilla extract
+ 2 figs
+ 2 c baby spinach

Instructions:

1. Soak the almonds overnight in the liquid if desired.
2. Grind the almonds.
3. Add the water if you did not soak the almonds, and the ice.
4. Add the pear, vanilla extract, and figs.
5. Add the baby spinach.
6. Blend at the highest speed for 30-45 seconds.

Nutrition Facts

Serving Size 1 Serving
% Based on 2000 Calorie Diet

Per Serving	% Daily Value
Calories 359	18.0%
Calories from Fat 135	
Total Fat 15.0g	23%
Saturated Fat 1.2g	6%
Cholesterol 0mg	0%
Sodium 68mg	3%
Potassium 970mg	28%
Carbohydrates 54.0g	18%
Dietary Fiber 12.9g	52%
Sugars 33.5g	
Protein 9.5g	
Vitamin A 113%	Vitamin C 39%
Calcium 22%	Iron 21%

This green smoothie has no cholesterol and is low in saturated fat and sodium. It is high in dietary fiber, manganese, magnesium, vitamin A, and vitamin C.

Kale Citrus Green Smoothie

Ingredients:
+ 1 c water
+ 1 c almond milk
+ 1 c papaya cubes frozen
+ 1 orange, peeled without seeds
+ ½ lime, peeled
+ 2 c kale

Instructions:
1. Add the liquid base in the blender first.
2. Add the orange and papaya.
3. Add the kale and lime.
4. Blend at the highest speed for 30-45 seconds.

Nutrition Facts

Serving Size 1 Serving
% Based on 2000 Calorie Diet

Per Serving	% Daily Value
Calories 379	19.0%
Calories from Fat 133	
Total Fat 14.8g	23%
Saturated Fat 1.2g	6%
Cholesterol 0mg	0%
Sodium 77mg	3%
Potassium 1465mg	42%
Carbohydrates 57.4g	19%
Dietary Fiber 12.5g	50%
Sugars 29.7g	
Protein 12.4g	
Vitamin A 448%	Vitamin C 578%
Calcium 37%	Iron 21%

This green smoothie has no cholesterol and is low in saturated fat and sodium. It is high in dietary fiber, manganese, magnesium, potassium, vitamin A, and vitamin C.

Berry Berry Goji Berries Green Smoothie

Ingredients:
- 2 c water
- 1 c frozen mixed berries
- 2 tbsp. goji berries
- ½ scoop protein powder
- 2 tbsp. cacao powder
- 2 c spinach

Instructions:
1. Add the liquid base first.
2. Add the goji berries and mixed berries.
3. Add the cacao powder and protein powder.
4. Add the baby spinach.
5. Blend at the highest speed for 30-45 seconds.

Nutrition Facts

Serving Size 1 Serving
% Based on 2000 Calorie Diet

Per Serving	% Daily Value
Calories 259	13.0%
Calories from Fat 43	
Total Fat 4.8g	7%
Saturated Fat 1.8g	9%
Cholesterol 32mg	11%
Sodium 89mg	4%
Potassium 607mg	17%
Carbohydrates 43.2g	14%
Dietary Fiber 11.5g	46%
Sugars 25.7g	
Protein 16.5g	
Vitamin A 115%	Vitamin C 102%
Calcium 16%	Iron 68%

This green smoothie is low in sodium. It is high in dietary fiber, iron, vitamin A, and vitamin C.

Kiwi Mango Green Smoothie

Ingredients:

- 1 oz. almonds raw or roasted (no salt)
- 1 c water
- 1 c unsweetened coconut water
- 10-15 mint leaves
- 2 kiwi fruit peeled
- 1 mango cubed and frozen
- 2 c kale

Instructions:

1. Soak the almonds overnight in the water, if desired.
2. Grind the almonds and add the liquid.
3. Add the mango, kiwi fruit, and mint leaves.
4. Add the kale.
5. Blend at the highest speed for 30-45 seconds.

Nutrition Facts

Serving Size 1 Serving
% Based on 2000 Calorie Diet

Per Serving	% Daily Value
Calories 323	16.1%
Calories from Fat 135	
Total Fat 15.0g	23%
Saturated Fat 1.1g	5%
Cholesterol 0mg	0%
Sodium 63mg	3%
Potassium 1340mg	38%
Carbohydrates 42.4g	14%
Dietary Fiber 10.1g	40%
Sugars 14.9g	
Protein 11.7g	
Vitamin A 415%	Vitamin C 503%
Calcium 31%	Iron 21%

This green smoothie has no cholesterol and is low in sodium. It is high in dietary fiber, manganese, magnesium, potassium, vitamin A, and vitamin C.

Plum Blackberry Green Smoothie

Ingredients:
- 1 c soy milk
- 1 c water
- 1 c frozen blackberries
- 2 pitted black plums (or pluots)
- 1 tbsp. chia seeds (soaked for 5-10 minutes)
- 2 c collard leaves

Instructions:
1. Add the liquid base in the blender first.
2. Add the plums, blackberries, & chia seeds.
3. Add the collard leaves.
4. Blend at the highest speed for 30-45 seconds.

Nutrition Facts

Serving Size 1 Serving
% Based on 2000 Calorie Diet

Per Serving	% Daily Value
Calories 344	17.2%
Calories from Fat 90	
Total Fat 10.0g	15%
Saturated Fat 1.1g	5%
Cholesterol 0mg	0%
Sodium 188mg	8%
Potassium 719mg	21%
Carbohydrates 48.9g	16%
Dietary Fiber 19.0g	76%
Sugars 30.8g	
Protein 15.7g	
Vitamin A 111%	Vitamin C 115%
Calcium 28%	Iron 22%

This green smoothie has no cholesterol and is low in saturated fat. It is high in dietary fiber, manganese, magnesium, vitamin A, and vitamin C.

Plum Banana Green Smoothie

Ingredients:
- 1 oz. hazelnuts raw or roasted (no salt)
- 2 c water
- 2 pitted black plums (or pluots)
- 1 frozen banana
- 2 stalks celery chopped and frozen
- 2 c baby spinach

Instructions:
1. Soak the nuts overnight if desired.
2. Grind the nuts and add the liquid.
3. Add the banana, plums, and celery.
4. Add the spinach.
5. Blend at the highest speed for 30-45 seconds.

Nutrition Facts

Serving Size 1 Serving
% Based on 2000 Calorie Diet

Per Serving	% Daily Value
Calories 364	18.2%
Calories from Fat 161	
Total Fat 17.9g	28%
Saturated Fat 1.5g	7%
Cholesterol 0mg	0%
Sodium 86mg	4%
Potassium 1042mg	30%
Carbohydrates 49.7g	17%
Dietary Fiber 9.4g	38%
Sugars 29.5g	
Protein 8.4g	
Vitamin A 126%	Vitamin C 72%
Calcium 12%	Iron 21%

This green smoothie has no cholesterol and is low in sodium and saturated fat. It is high in dietary fiber, manganese, vitamin A, and vitamin C.

Message from the Author

Nothing tickles me more than when I hear from one of my readers. I love reading their stories of challenges and successes. Sometimes they even let me know when they find a typo in one of my books (for which am eternally grateful)! My writing is a work in progress. If there is something you think I can do to make this book a better experience for other readers, let me know about it. You can connect with me by email at francesca@brightideaseditoria.com, via twitter at @francescafoodie, or on my Facebook page.

If you'd like to help other readers decide if this book is for them, I'd be grateful if you could take a moment and post a sentence or two as a review on Amazon. Reader comments are the most powerful and unbiased way for others to determine which books should make the short list for their next read. And I promise I'll read every word.

Cheers,

Francesca

May I Suggest...

Other books by Francesca DiMarco

The Mediterranean Diet Cookbook for Beginners...who Love to Eat, with 75 Authentic Recipes by Executive Chef Kostas Magoulas

Other books published by Bright Ideas Editoria Ltd.
By Ryan J. S. Martin

Magnesium Deficiency: Weight Loss, Heart Disease and Depression, 13 Ways that Curing Your Magnesium Deficiency Can Rejuvenate Your Body

10,000 Steps: Walking for Weight Loss, Walking for Health: A Turn by Turn Roadmap

The Vitamin D Cure: 8 Surprising Ways Curing Your Vitamin D Deficiency Can Revitalize Your Health, Prevent Heart Disease and Cancer, and Help You Lose Weight

FREE DOWNLOAD

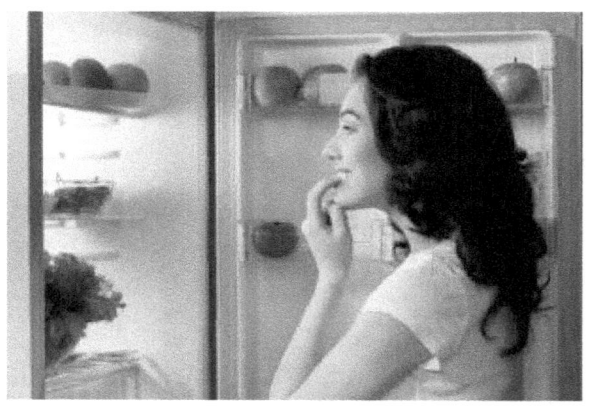

As a thank you for purchasing this book, I've created a free report full of healthy snack ideas, just for you!

FREE REPORT REVEALS 10 SCRUMPTIOUS SNACKS UNDER 200 CALORIES

"Smash the hangries with these skinny snacks (if your kids don't eat them first)"

You can download the free report at
http://editoria.leadpages.net/snacks/